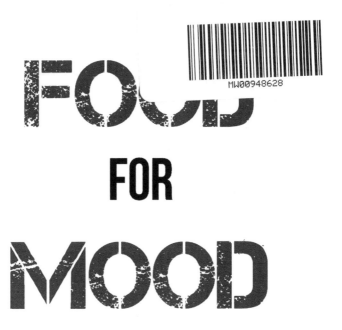

FOR

MOOD

DIETARY AND LIFESTYLE INTERVENTIONS FOR ANXIETY, DEPRESSION, AND OTHER MOOD DISORDERS

BY: **MATT STONE**

www.180degreehealth.com

Published by Archangel Ink
ISBN: 1505326362
ISBN-13: 978-1505326369

Table of Contents

Introduction

Once upon a time, I wrote a book with an equally simplistic, rhyming title. It was called *Eat for Heat*, and it was released on December 1, 2012. About two years ago.

Pretty amazing story so far I know. Riveting. Try not to fall off of your seat.

The release of that book was a big deal. It was the first book I had published in over a year (for me, that's a long time), and it was the first time I had published a book on Amazon. The book did spectacularly well, and the few thousand or so people that followed my blog religiously at the time were quite pleased to see their favorite blogger tearing up the bestseller charts over on Amazon. They bought it and bought it and bought it until it reached the top 100 books in all of the Kindle store.

More importantly, as it pertains to the subject of this book, I encouraged my peeps to write reviews to help let people know that my book was legit despite how strange and contradictory its contents were. And they did. Within a few days they had written nearly 100, heartfelt, long-winded reviews talking about how effing hilarious I am and sharing their personal experiences with implementing the information in the book as well as other stuff I'd been putting out for years prior.

Among those reviews, something really stood out. Again and again there were mentions of anxiety, specifically, being relieved when applying the tactics I discussed. It made sense as to why. The goal of the tactics I recommended were to minimize stress hormones, putting the body into a relaxed, parasympathetic-dominant state. This state of low stress, physical relaxation, and so forth is obviously very conducive to quieting down anxiety, irritability, aggression, and other unpleasant emotions. But why? That, among other mood-related discussions, will be the primary focus of this book.

Who am I to write a book about such matters? Well I've been studied in 17 different countries by dozens of research teams, and it's been conclusively shown that I'm the happiest, sanest, most stable human being on earth. Even just a cursory glance at my charts from a recent EEG performed by Johnny Hopkins shows clearly how happy I am:

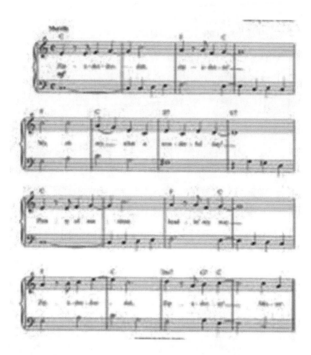

Researchers were immediately baffled at what they saw, as this scan so clearly shows what appears to be sheet music. Upon close examination and review by a panel of musicians at Juilliard, it was revealed that this actually could be translated into music that includes lyrics, although the team of linguists have been unable to establish what language it is derived from. So far all they have managed to capture is what, to a modern ear, sounds like jibberish. It goes…

"Zip a dee doo dah, zip a dee ay."

Yeah, I'm not sure what it means either, but they feel confident that it displays exceptional happiness that has yet to be documented by any of the world's top research organizations.

No, no. I'm not really any happier than anyone else. In fact, I'm a pretty miserable, conceited, reclusive bastard with a tendency to take out frustrations on inanimate objects like a crazy person. I fit the typical profile of a writer to the letter. My capacity for processing and dealing with emotions isn't anything to be marveled. I'm not talking about attaining general happiness.

That's not the point or purpose of this book really. Nor is it within the scope of this book to talk about anything that could be chalked up to circumstances a person might find themselves in. Hey, sometimes you're going to perceive life as shitty no matter who you are or how fabulous your life is compared to others.

My eFriend Thomas said it best when he stated (paraphrasing):

"If you're not at least a little depressed living in today's modern world, there's probably something really wrong with you."

But what I want to shed light on is the type of pathology where anger, agitation, anxiety, panic, and soul-sucking depression seem to come out of nowhere—arising more as physical sensations that don't seem to have much circumstantial basis. And this kind of emotional instability usually has a lot less to do with circumstances and mindset and a lot more to do with physical phenomena. I'm talking about cascades of hormones and neurotransmitters that occur when the body is in a stressful state. Physical stress puts the mind in a state of mental stress, and intense emotions can ensue for no apparent rhyme or reason. Also, in a compromised physical state, our reaction to certain people, events, and circumstances as well as the thinking patterns that emerge, are distinctly different.

We've all experienced going irrationally and unjustifiably apeshit over something tiny. Likewise, most of us have had the experience of having something truly terrible happen but having states of complete and total happiness and contentedness in the face of circumstances that would seem to warrant strong, negative emotions. In my extensive experience with being in a variety of physical states induced by ridiculous dietary and lifestyle experiments, I think much of this emotional rollercoaster ride that we know as life can be contained within much tighter boundaries of sanity and rationality. Or, if we do things that are counterproductive to our own health and biochemical stability, we experience peaks and valleys that are much more likely to go beyond the boundaries of acceptability.

In this book I hope to deliver some tools that can help you become more cognizant of your physiological state in maintaining greater emotional stability. For some, the information in this book will be outrageously helpful. I've dealt with hundreds of people over the years to know that what I will be discussing has great power for individuals in need of such interventions. I know the power myself, as I truly cannot control my emotions when my physical needs are not abundantly met. I go, as the movie character Clifford says, "nutty nuts."

For others, this information won't be particularly helpful. Please know that I'm not intending to write the seminal work to be used by all human beings as the eternal key to happiness. A book like that could never conceivably exist, so please do me and you both a favor by not treating it as such.

The title, *Food for Mood*, is also a little inaccurate. But who cares about accuracy really? It rhymes. That's all that really matters in life.

Such a title suggests that the book will be about food, and it really won't be. The fact that being hungry and underfed can lead to radical changes in one's emotional state is hardly a groundbreaking, book-worthy subject. Even the marketing team for Snickers knows that. While food can play an important role in maintaining the physiological stability that can lend itself to greater emotional stability in most individuals, it's but one tool. We'll be discussing lots of tools: Justin Bieber, Pat Robinson, Dr. Oz. Alright, not those kind of tools. Different ones.

Okay, I suppose we better get started now. First, let me briefly rant about emotions. They are kind of ridiculous when you really think about it.

Under the Influence of Emotion

People tend to take their emotions so seriously. Please don't. You'll always be at a disadvantage when you buy into your emotions as having great relevance. In many cases, your emotions are just a temporary distraction from rational thought. While they can certainly be used as tools when used intelligently, it is a rare individual who can actually do something intelligent when under the influence of emotion. If you define intelligent thought as balanced, broad-spectrum, mature thinking—emotion could even be defined as a temporary lapse in intelligence.

Emotions, by their simplest definition, are something we experience when we perceive something as being more negative than positive or more positive than negative. In other words, when our thoughts and perceptions are unbalanced, emotions arise. The stronger the imbalance between positive and negative, the stronger the emotional state. Since we are constantly thinking and perceiving, we are bound to be riding an emotional rollercoaster throughout our lives. We can have temporary moments of feeling "above our emotions" or enlightened somehow, but, humans that we are, our hard-wiring ensures that we continually work our way into unbalanced states and experience a symphony of emotions as a result.

Please don't fight emotions either. All we are seeking to do here is to turn down the volume of this emotional orchestra to something a little more reasonable. The point of doing that is to merely help us stay on track and stay focused on what we really want to be doing with our lives. More importantly, we can be confident that no one will upload a video of us on YouTube freaking out over something trivial, which may or may not include attempts to rectally insert a remote control in our temporary state of irrationality.

https://www.youtube.com/watch?v=YersIyzsOpc

What I'm saying is that we're going to experience emotion even though emotion itself is kinda dumb. And when we do, we should do our best not to take it all that seriously—not that seriously in ourselves or that seriously in that of others. Emotions come and go. They are temporary and transient and not something that should be taken very seriously and analyzed to pieces in addition to the absurdity of experiencing them. I'm not just talking about negative emotions either, as overly positive emotions are just as dangerous and irrational— often leading to rash, unintelligent decisions and feelings of mild depression and dissatisfaction the moment we come down from the high.

Before we get started, let's just be real about emotions. What's the most ridiculous thing you've ever done when under the influence of a strong emotion? And what was the trigger for that emotional outburst? Let me tell you—I've always been a pretty intense person. My emotions are not something to fool around with. And when I start doing something physiologically compromising, watch out. The embarrassing things that I've done in highly emotional states are too voluminous to mention, but I will mention a few just to hopefully make you feel a little bit more normal about who you are and what you've done.

For starters, let me just say that technology is my nemesis. Most people have a lot of built up emotional baggage with their exes, their siblings, their parents. People that picked on them in high school. Not me. It's those damn gadgets. Everything I do is pretty much internet based, so that means not only do I have a vast assortment of gadgetry that could annoy me at any given moment, but I also have server issues, autoresponder issues, affiliate software, mass payments, audio editing issues, and a seemingly bottomless list of things that could go wrong. And something always does. Especially Skype. Damn you Skype!

When it does, who knows what my reaction might be. Funnily enough, I'm writing on a brand new keyboard because I smashed my last one into about 80 pieces the week before I started writing this book over some technology-related fiasco. I've broken Venetian blinds. I've thrown a trash can full of chicken bones across the house, breaking the trash can and turning half the living room into what smelled and felt like chicken vomit. And recently a server issue made me look like such a fool, ruined important business connections of mine, tarnished my reputation, and I was so powerless to fix it, that I actually started playing out suicide scenarios in my head. Don't worry, I could never commit suicide. I'm way too much of a pussy to ever do something like that. I can barely ride rollercoasters anymore. Just being honest. We all have some pretty insane thoughts creep in from time to time if we're being honest.

Remove emotion though, and my thinking is quite fair and balanced. I'm quite thankful for modern technology, which has afforded me the ability to totally live the dream of achieving complete departure from location-based work. I can go anywhere whenever I want. I don't own an alarm clock. I work (or don't work) my own hours. I make money all night long while I sleep.

There are relationships, too. Wow do we do some stupid things in our relationships. It's like we save our most juvenile behavior for those we love the most. I once banged my head on a toilet seat I was so upset about some relationship quarrel (don't even remember what it was about). Not quite sure what I was trying to achieve by that. Pretty funny in retrospect. Matt the human plunger with bad aim.

But none of it compares to the sick, deranged emotions I experienced when I was at the low point of meeting my physiological needs. Up and down I rode on the mother of all rollercoasters between some sort of spiritual ecstasy and complete depression and rage. Thinking back to the time I starved myself down to the point of having veins popping out my abs, I can see it all crystal clear even though experiencing it felt like a blur. It came to a climax when I started shouting at a tent in the presence of others while out camping, seeing myself act like a complete lunatic but being completely unable to tap into my logical mind and regain control.

I bring all this up to help us all lighten up a bit. We do strange things to one another when under the influence of emotion. And other people do strange things to us. Funny things. Hurtful things. Sometimes even violent things. Sucks that we have to spend so much of our lives burdened with the temporary insanity of emotion. Sometimes they can be fun. Music and movies wouldn't be much fun if we didn't have emotions. We'd be pretty lousy lovers as well. Emotions are not all bad. Hey, don't get emotional about your emotions!

We're going to feel emotion, and emotions are important to the human experience. But do we really need to experience such great extremes and intensities of emotion? Do we need to experience more emotion than we already do? Or should we investigate some ways to support our mental and emotional stability by keeping our physiology more stable with a variety of tactics?

That's where we're headed next. First we'll explore the anatomy of my favorite emotion to discuss, what I've found to be the easiest to resolve, and the original inspiration for writing this book: anxiety.

Anxiety

Interestingly, I've never really experienced any severe degree of anxiety. For me personally, it's just not a go-to emotion. I'm much more likely to feel bummed out or irritable and angry when I'm off kilter. Anxiety tends to be more of a perceived fear of something out in the future, and, many times to my detriment, I'm always delusionally optimistic about the future. I don't worry. I'm all Bobby McFerrin when it comes to stuff like that. So it's kind of interesting that I've taken an interest in anxiety specifically. It's really just a matter of several things converging, the most significant of which is having lots of people plagued with anxiety tell me how much less of it they experienced after doing a few things to stimulate their metabolisms and lower their stress levels.

The Autonomic Nervous System

First let's take a simple look at the nervous system. While there are many criminally oversimplified generalizations out there about the sympathetic and parasympathetic nervous systems (together forming the autonomic nervous system), and I've been convicted many times of the crime of oversimplification, the basic working understanding of it is effective enough to provide a decent mental framework for what they are. The sympathetic nervous system is more of the active side of the nervous system, as opposed to its drowsy counterpart, the parasympathetic nervous system.

Let's say you're working on a project. Or you're concentrating while writing an email to an important colleague. Or you're out on a jog or in the middle of a strenuous workout. All of these things are generally done with the sympathetic nervous system active and the parasympathetic nervous system relatively inactive in comparison.

Your parasympathetic nervous system tends to predominate when you're relaxed, lying down, just coming out of a Jacuzzi, asleep, or feeling the familiar sensation of post-meal drowsiness after a big feast.

Coinciding with these two contrasting states of the nervous system are behavioral and thought tendencies. You're unlikely to have a panic attack right after a slice of cheesecake or getting a massage. But early in the morning while rushing out the door on a skimpy breakfast, watch out.

Those are more moment to moment diurnal fluctuations for the most part however, and isn't something that we should probably dwell on too much. Rather, we need to take a look at what could be considered more chronic elevation of the sympathetic nervous system and/or pathologically dynamic fluctuations.

With chronic sympathetic dominance, instead of the normal peaks and valleys in nervous system activity throughout the day—with the sympathetic and parasympathetic nervous systems seesawing up and down—many experience a tendency to spend more time in the sympathetic-dominant state, and perhaps experience very big spikes that lead to acute anxiety events one or more times per day.

Others still are not chronically in the sympathetic-dominant state but still suffer extreme anxiety and panic attacks frequently. In this scenario, a person is usually experiencing the normal fluctuations between high and low sympathetic nervous system dominance, but those fluctuations are pathologically dramatic. In other words, all of the same emotions and physical states are experienced just like a normal person, but the peaks and valleys are much stronger. This is more of a bipolar type of pattern, but it's not necessarily repeated bouts of happy and sad as is seen in a more classic case of bipolar disorder. Rather, it's more of repeated bouts of extremes of energy—going from manic, fidgety, hyperventilation, insomnia, etc. to extreme fatigue. And coinciding with those extreme peaks and valleys are often extremes of emotion—either super hyper and excited paired with groggy and mopey or anxiety interspersed with depression.

Thus, when dealing with anxiety I really think there are two distinct physiological/psychological profile types: constant and intermittent.

Firstly, let's talk about constant and chronic sympathetic nervous system hyperactivity and the increased tendency towards anxiety and manic behavior.

To be sure, this tendency is without a doubt hereditary—at least in part. Pretty much everything that we physiologically or emotionally experience is hereditary to some extent. But this hereditary tendency can be intensified or subdued depending on the infinite number of factors that comprise life.

Metabolic Rate and Anxiety

It's at this point that my work in metabolism and stress hormone production comes into play, as a low metabolic rate works to constantly suppress the activity of the parasympathetic nervous system—leading to a chronic elevation of stress hormones.

http://www.ncbi.nlm.nih.gov/pubmed/2254712

Kind of an oversimplification again, as the stress cascade probably begins in the pituitary where the secretion of thyroid-stimulating hormone originates, elevated levels of which are synonymous with both hypothyroidism and high cortisol levels (cortisol is the primary "stress hormone").

http://www.ncbi.nlm.nih.gov/pmc/articles/PMC3520819/

I believe this works both ways, as many biological systems do—chronic stress hormone elevation can lead to a low metabolic rate just as low metabolic rate leads to chronic stress hormone elevation. The question is, why?

Gee, I'm glad you asked. This is the whole geekfest part I've been waiting to write. I won't go off too much, but I think it's both interesting and empowering for people with any kind of mood disorder to realize that it's not just "in their head." Nothing is ever just "in your head" I assure you. There are endless physiological reasons why emotions can become debilitatingly strong, and gaining a better understanding of how your body works can be a major key in achieving success in your attempts to better yourself.

What we're talking about here are basically polarities of physical function that can lead to polarities of emotion. Consider thyroid (representing metabolic rate), to be the primary representative of the parasympathetic nervous system (chillin'), while cortisol can be considered the primary representative of the sympathetic nervous system (anxious). When one goes up, the other goes down—generally-speaking.

So take the most classic example into account that also happens to be what I find to be the most common exacerbator (chuckle) of anxiety and panic attacks—dieting. Dieting lowers thyroid and raises cortisol with near 100% consistency. It's very simple physiology. Deprive the body of energy, and it perceives this as a great stress, lowering resting metabolic rate to preserve energy. This is predominantly controlled by the fat tissue itself. As fat tissue decreases during forced calorie deficit, leptin falls, which decreases metabolic rate. Metabolic rate stays suppressed until body fat reserves are replenished to prior levels plus interest.

While there is an endless mountain of false hype out there about how dieting and exercise and weight loss via a forced, controlled calorie deficit are going to make you "feel super fantastic and fabulous," this just isn't reality. You might feel good about how you look. You might even temporarily feel a little buzz from the increase in stress hormones (the "catecholamine honeymoon" as I'm known for dubbing this phenomenon), but overall you're working very hard against your physiology.

If you push hard enough, and you have a tendency towards anxiety, get ready to feel a lot more of it. This is because stress hormones start to rise as metabolic rate falls, and the body starts to spend more time in a sympathetic-dominant state. That rock opera of emotions often emerges, dominated by manic thoughts, anxiety, and agitation—among other strange things. The insomnia that often accompanies it (hard to sleep with extra cortisol and adrenaline surging through your veins, which are diuretic to boot) doesn't help much either.

So the most basic piece of useful information you'll get here, and the backbone of the "food for mood" concept, is to first and foremost quit dieting in just about every form. Extremes of macronutrient restriction such as very low-carb dieting, calorie restriction, intermittent fasting, juice fasting/cleansing, strict veganism, and raw foodism are but a short list of diets that will likely exacerbate anxiety issues and mood instability in general. This also holds true even when one of the various forms of eating just mentioned causes a dramatic improvement to your mood in the short-term. Even a well-intentioned attempt to pursue "healthy eating" can lead to inadvertent failure to consume adequate calories, metabolic downregulation, and a worsening of anxiety.

If you suffer from anxiety and panic attacks specifically, and you have a history of dieting or intentionally restricting food or undereating, the very first thing you should do before exploring any other therapies, treatments, or tactics is to consistently eat an adequate number of calories every single day without interruption. Unfortunately, quantifying exactly how many calories one needs to eat to get the proper results is nearly impossible. Nor do most people find counting calories to be very practical. Therefore, the first step is to merely eat to fullness of foods that sound appealing to you every time you feel hungry. That usually ensures adequate calorie consumption, and will be enough for many to experience significantly lessened anxiety.

Just eating to appetite doesn't work for everyone though. Before giving up on the potential of using something as simple as eating enough as a therapeutic intervention, try tracking your calories more closely. I have used formulas in the past for the purposes of "refeeding," or intentionally eating extra calories in an attempt to raise metabolic rate for those who need to, but they still lacked precision. I suggest using a basal metabolic rate calculator online, entering your estimated weight with very little extra body fat, and multiplying your result by 1.5 if you're totally sedentary. If you're physically active, you'll need more—perhaps a lot more.

For example, using the calculator at this website, http://www.calculator.net/bmr-calculator.html, my basal metabolic rate is calculated at 1,828. That's an estimation with normal metabolic function if I were in a coma. But even lying in bed and thinking about stuff, especially the stuff I think about, will increase your daily caloric expenditure. Normal daily activities like doing a few household chores, going to work, running a few errands, and walking up an occasional flight of stairs will bring it up closer to 1.5 times your basal metabolic rate.

Thus, I multiply 1,828 by 1.5 to get 2,742.

I know personally that's a little low for me, even when completely sedentary (my body temperature and pulse rate run slightly lower at that calorie intake, which are signs of reduced metabolic rate), but it's not too far off. I like to go on long walks several days per week and do a little resistance training here and there, and although I don't track calories at all, I would estimate that I'm consistently in the 3,000-3,500 calorie range depending on physical activity levels. My 9-year old daughter eats more than 2.0 times her BMR calculation daily. So consider the BMR figure multiplied by 1.5 *to be an absolute minimum number of calories you should ingest daily whether you are physically active or not.*

MINIMUM!

Sorry for yelling. Many people need the volume to be turned up to hear this though, as we are conditioned to believe that calories are inherently bad, and the fewer of them we eat the better. I assure you that if you are unable to eat that many calories daily and stay weight stable, your metabolic rate is poor, and if your metabolic rate is poor, you are or will be suffering health consequences from it—possibly including a mood disorder like anxiety.

Correcting a low metabolism isn't always a simple matter of eating an adequate amount of food, but it often is. Increasing a low metabolism isn't always sufficient to improve or resolve anxiety, but it often is. We're not talking about a panacea here. We're talking about a reasonable place to start—because one should always start with the simplest solution and work up from there if it's not effective. If you have anxiety, the first thing you should try is eating more, especially if you have reason to suspect that you've been chronically failing to consume the amount of calories specified above.

Now let's talk a little bit more about metabolic rate and the anatomy of anxiety for more connections and more therapeutic interventions you can add for success. Even if you don't suffer from anxiety, it's very interesting stuff.

Carbon Dioxide

We're all familiar with the classic movie scene of someone having a panic attack and breathing into a paper sack to calm down. While it's cliché, there are tremendous physiology lessons here.

First of all, carbon dioxide is a very metabolism-stimulating gas. Likewise (the whole two-way street thing again), a rise in metabolic rate will increase carbon dioxide levels in the body. Stress can cause hyperventilation, which creates a rapid lowering of carbon dioxide, which initializes a scary cascade—as the more you hyperventilate the more you panic and the more you panic or feel anxious the more you hyperventilate. But stopping the excessive loss of carbon dioxide from excessive breathing immediately helps to calm the nervous system and relieve anxiety. Carbon dioxide is that powerful, and the interesting thing is *that as metabolic rate falls, carbon dioxide levels decrease, making people a lot more prone to anxiety.*

For a more elegant discussion on carbon dioxide, read Ray Peat's article on carbon dioxide at http://raypeat.com/articles/articles/protective-co2-aging.shtml or some of the work of Danny Roddy.

Simply put, raise metabolic rate, become less anxiety prone. Decrease metabolic rate, become more anxiety prone. It's that simple. And much of it has to do with carbon dioxide for reasons that are far too vast to explore here. It gets to the root of cellular energy metabolism and respiration at its foundation.

Eating to raise metabolic rate aside, it's also possible, through various relaxation and breathing techniques, to increase metabolic rate and reduce anxiety tendencies. This is true both in the acute sense and in the chronic sense.

In acute anxiety events, you don't necessarily have to breathe into a paper sack, although you could, but bringing focus to your breath and doing everything in your power to slow your rate of breathing to a normal, relaxed pace can instantly relieve an anxiety attack. You could even try gently holding your breath to restore carbon dioxide levels to normal and bring about a system-wide calming effect to the sympathetic nervous system. The only problem with this is that it is a lot easier said than done. It's like telling a little leaguer to get up there and "hit the ball." A better analogy might be telling someone in a fit of rage to have a warm bath with rose petals and a cup of chamomile tea. I might cut a bitch if he/she gave me this advice in the middle of a webhosting outage.

And so, it's probably more appropriate to turn our focus to the prevention of anxiety attacks, and breathing exercises that aim to increase carbon dioxide levels can be very useful—not just for anxiety prevention but general health.

I won't even pretend to be an expert on this. I've never done anything close to a breathing exercise in my life. When I've attempted to do some, I gave up in under two minutes. If doing breathing exercises sounds like torture to you, equal or greater to the torture of experiencing bouts of anxiety, I can relate. But some swear by it, the basis for why it is effective is sound, and it should be voiced in any conversation about anxiety—if only to better understand how our bodies function and get closer to the root of the problem.

There is a lot of confusion about what constitutes proper breathing. There are also all kinds of breathing methods out there—some completely and totally at odds with retaining higher levels of carbon dioxide and thus stifling anxiety. Lemme tell ya a little story.

Over a decade ago before I knew squat about diddley, my girlfriend at the time had minor anxiety tendencies. In certain situations it was an emotion that she gravitated towards. Nothing that could be called a mood disorder, abnormal, or pathological.

She was a very curious explorer of health ideas. A little too curious if you catch my drift (aren't we all?). She attended some kind of breathwork hippie pow-wow. You know those. I don't remember the name of this sacred, consciousness-raising baloney, but it involved hyperventilating. For some, hyperventilation might make them feel funny. For my girlfriend, some very strange things happened that weren't so funny. She felt an extreme bout of anxiety and had her hands and other muscles start to cramp up. These are, of course, symptoms of hyperventilation, and it's not a good thing. The hippies had no idea what went wrong because they obviously had no earthly idea what they were doing, or they wouldn't have been practicing their idiotic form of breathwork in the first place. I didn't get any of that then, but I get it with crystal clarity now.

The point of the story is that any type of breathing exercise to raise metabolic rate, increase carbon dioxide levels, lower internal stress hormone production, and improve anxiety, should be focused on breathing less, not more. Breaths should be more shallow, not deeper (the whole "take a deep breath" to calm down thing is totally backwards). Basically, you want your breathing to be extremely calm just as you might breathe when totally relaxed. I mean, do you take huge audible breaths when you're relaxed with your chest cavity expanding way out? I hope not. You're a total weirdo if you do.

The most common breathing method with goals aligned with what we're trying to accomplish in a pro-metabolic, anti-anxiety sense, is the Buteyko Method. The Buteyko Method is named after Konstantin Pavlovich Buteyko, who is best known for parachuting into a small rural town with some comrades of his and taking the citizens hostage in 1984. He was later shot down by Patrick Swayze. Serves him right for shooting a bunch of holes into Jennifer Grey in that helicopter ambush. Poor little thing.

Okay, maybe that wasn't Konstantin Buteyko, and maybe that was, in fact, *Red Dawn*. I have a reputation to uphold when it comes to 80's movie references. And I'd say I pretty much hit that out of the park like Andre Dawson in 1987. Incidentally, Andre feels the same way about pitches outside of the strike zone as I do about malfunctioning electronics. https://www.youtube.com/watch?v=oAKkHxkkCyA

Buteyko breathing involves very slow, shallow breathing with the intent of extending what is referred to as the "control pause," or the amount of time one comfortably can hold their breath without having to hyperventilate afterwards to compensate for the oxygen shortage. While the Buteyko breathing movement can be quite cultish and extreme, working with practitioners to learn this breathing method outrageously expensive, and the practice of doing it a far cry from enjoyable, it can be an effective supplement to other metabolism-stimulating, stress-reducing tactics. For some honest and inexpensive discussion on proper breathing, I recommend the book *Breathe* by Joey Lott.

Hydration and Electrolytes

As I'm sure you've heard countless other places, it's very important to drink your body weight in pounds in fluid ounces each day and consume a ton of potassium. Salt is bad for you, so stay away from that nasty stuff!

Aside from that brief, facetious paragraph, you won't hear that in this place. Similar to the upside down world of breathing exercises that perform the exact opposite of the desired effect, the beliefs about hydration and electrolytes are completely upside down, too. It's weird, as one of the greatest medical interventions in history has been the intravenous administration of saline solution, with the equivalent of 13 ½ medium-sized orders of French fries worth of salt added to each liter of it. Doctors often administer more than one liter in a matter of hours, with amazing benefits.

Yet down the hall in "Dietary" they are preparing bland food with hardly any salt in it, as if ingesting salt orally is bad and can only be beneficial when injected directly into the blood. Once when my elderly grandfather was in the hospital they actually had him hooked up to a bag of saline solution and brought him a plate of low sodium food prescribed by the dietician on staff. Now that's comedy. In case you ever wondered if the medical industry at large was confused, now you have proof. Actually, it appears the medical industry is doing alright. It's the Nutritionistas (intentional spelling) that are confused. Come to think of it, the problem is not that they are confused, it's that they aren't confused. How can you be certain about something that there are few if any definitive answers about? But I digress.

Lemme tell ya another story about the ex-girlfriend with tendencies towards anxiety…

I have this terrible habit of being buddy buddy with all of my exes. It's awful. Fortunately, I was never that much of a playboy, and the list of my ex-girlfriends is in the single digits. But I swear I'm in close communication with nearly all of them.

I have so little boundaries when it comes to my exes that I actually tested the concentration of her urine. Yeah, I had her pee in a cup, and then I ran some little tests on it. It was pretty pale, with a brix just above 1.0 if I recall. At the time, despite taking a lot of proactive measures on the psychological front to quell her anxiety, she was getting hit hard almost daily in the mid-morning hours. The timing here has to do with daily hormonal fluctuations as well as what some incorrectly call "low blood sugar," both of which we'll briefly discuss in a later section.

Getting back to the story, I told her to simply stop drinking so much water, especially in the morning. I knew how obsessed she was with her water. We had done all kinds of dumb new age things together like write happy words on our five-gallon water jug a la that Japanese guy. Plus, she always carried around a bottle of water everywhere she went.

Within days the anxiety was gone.

Here's what's going on...

Think back to the two-way street of hyperventilation and anxiety. Anxiety induces hyperventilation, but hyperventilation also induces anxiety. The same is true of urine. When we experience anxiety and fear, we have a tendency to "pee our pants." The urge to urinate is very strong, urine concentration falls (even without drinking anything), and frequent urination often ensues.

In the same two-way fashion, but by drinking too many fluids, it is possible to induce anxiety. Those with a low metabolism also have a lot less of a buffer for fluids, with even small amounts of water "going right through them." That is another key factor involved in urine concentration and what I would call "fluid tolerance" or "water threshold." Daily rhythms are significant as well, as fluid tolerance is typically much lower in the first half of the day than the second half of the day, yet many people are consuming tons of watery stuff early in the day with very little salt: big glasses of lemon water, giant coffees, watery cereal or oatmeal, smoothies, fruit, fruit juice, and so on. This may be a perfectly healthy way for a healthy person to eat (I feel great eating that way in the morning now), but for someone with a low metabolism and problems with anxiety that often peaks in the mid-morning? No way.

This is yet another bone-headedly simple, seems like it couldn't possibly be helpful aspect of anxiety anatomy that any sufferer of the condition should be aware of and very attentive to. That's because it is phenomenally effective for the right person, with the ability to improve anxiety almost overnight in some. Even my own sister, who was urinating 0.0 brix urine several times per day (she actually tested her own… okay, I might have tested it once, too), had her anxiety and heart palpitations cease within a few days of normalizing her urine concentration.

Here's how to take advantage of this knowledge. It's very simple, so don't complicate it too much unless you find the following steps to be ineffective:

1. Make sure your urine is always nice and yellow, and strive to urinate roughly once every four hours during the day and none in the middle of the night.
2. If your urine becomes too clear, or you start urinating more frequently than that, adjust by eating more calorie-dense food that's also rich in carbohydrates (classic "junk food" works best, like pancakes, pizza, cheeseburgers, potato chips, and desserts—food for mood baby!), more salt, and drinking fewer fluids.
3. If your urine still won't get yellow, and your anxiety and frequent urination persists, stop drinking plain water completely for a while and switch to a high-sugar beverage like fruit juice or soda, consumed in small sips to just barely satisfy your thirst until color returns to your pee.

In an acute anxiety attack, you may also find relief by eating a dry, salty, carbohydrate-rich snack right away such as pretzels, crackers, dried fruit and jerky, or potato chips. In even more extreme situations, you may also find putting a large spoonful of white sugar and salt mixed together in about a 5-10:1 ratio under your tongue to provide quick relief.

Will this always work for all anxiety cases? Hell no! If it doesn't, that's a bummer, and you're going to have to keep digging. I hope you find your answers. But I know with certainty that some of the simple things discussed in this chapter regarding metabolic rate, calorie intake, breathing, hydration, and sodium intake can completely squash anxiety, even when circumstances present something anxiety-worthy.

If you need more information and guidance on metabolism, urine concentration and its relationship with nervous system activity, general food, fluid, and salt intake and more, you'll find way too much information in my other books—*Eat for Heat* in particular. Start here first though. Most people need more experimentation, not more information.

Other Common Sense Tactics

There are other things worth mentioning quickly that are also too simple and right under your nose to be ignored.

Get Warm

There is a close relationship between body coldness, metabolic rate, and stress hormone production. When your body or even just your extremities feel cold, which it often will if your metabolic rate is low, your stress hormones are higher and your propensity to experience anxiety is elevated. While you should be taking proactive measures to raise your metabolic rate, you can lend yourself a helping hand in both an acute and a chronic sense by keeping warm. Keep those hands and feet as warm as you can. And, if possible during an acute stress event, expose yourself to high heat. For most that will mean taking a nice warm bath or shower.

Exercise

Exercise is often touted as a stress reliever. While the body produces a lot of stress hormones during exercise, and the body is very much in a sympathetic-dominant state, it seems as if exercise replaces the mental stress as if physical stress is a healthier alternative to mental/emotional stress. Exercise can be used in acute stress events as a way to redirect your anxiety. It can also be used as a stress preventer, as if you go out and exhaust your adrenal glands so that they don't have enough juice to later produce feelings of anxiety and panic. Don't go crazy with the exercise, especially if you are in a vulnerable state with a low metabolic rate. Too much exercise will only make the root problem worse and will end up making you dependent on exhausting yourself daily to maintain a decent mood, which is far from ideal. But it has a role to play, and it can be used in concert with other tactics for greater mood stability.

Get Outside

Ever notice how your vision seems to get more focused when you consume a bunch of caffeine? It's as if your eyes widen and your pupils narrow. You may have also noticed the tendency to stare at things intensely that are at close range when very anxious or loaded up on stimulants. In typical two-way street fashion, it can induce stress to be staring at things at close range for long periods of time. This happens indoors, and it happens especially so when staring at a computer screen for hours on end. Going outdoors however, can instantly shift your mood and perspective, and I believe much of this has to do with the eyes. Not only is natural, bright light inherently de-stressing, but so is simply focusing your eyes on objects farther in the distance, and shifting your point of focus from near to far and back again rather than staying constantly fixated on something only a few feet from your nose. Likewise, closing your eyes completely has a similar, relaxing effect. Never forget the power of going outside if you suffer from mood problems of any kind. We'll discuss this more later, as this can be as powerful, or more powerful, than any other intervention for some.

This is just a short duh list. It could go on for a lot longer if I were so inclined, and include things like sex, sleep, lying down, massage, meditation, and much, much more. Obviously anything that is inherently de-stressing can be powerful therapy for anxiety. But we often forget or just plain overlook the simple solutions sitting right under our noses in favor of more exotic-sounding cures and potions. Please. Start with the easy, simple stuff. Always. With any health condition. There is more power in the basics than people realize. More sermons about the fundamentals await my children.

Hopefully that gives you some great new things to toy with if you are a sufferer of anxiety—tools to get to the root of the problem and eliminate the tendency to feel anxious in general, and tools to deal with acute bouts of anxiety and panic.

Next let's drift more into a general conversation about mood stability, as it's a rare individual that suffers from one and only one type of emotional malaise beyond what could be considered healthy. With some of the following insights, hopefully you'll be able to not only keep anxiety at bay, but keep your emotional state hugging much tighter to the midline of rationality day in and day out.

Mood Stability

I love the term "mood stability." Nearly everyone with any degree of emotional problems can enthusiastically nod their heads up and down when they hear the word "stable." Lack of stability is a common problem, and stable sounds like an awfully nice place to be. Not talking about the kind with hay and horse manure in it you wiseass.

It's next to impossible to maintain a perfectly stable mood. You'd have to be completely emotionless to pull that off I think. But I do think it's reasonable to expect to implement a handful of changes, assess your biofeedback, and bring about noticeable improvements. One thing I'd like to bring to your attention is our daily hormonal fluctuations.

Let's face it. We are not the same person with the same mood and mindset in the morning as we are midday and in the evening. A person with real mood stability problems can relate to this much better than someone without major issues in that area.

The most common pattern, although this is certainly not the only pattern, is to have a much higher proneness to mood swings in the mid-morning and mid-afternoon, and then feel absolutely fine after about 5pm. Hands and feet get warmer, urine gets more yellow, outlook gets more positive, laughter comes more easily, and patience is easier to tap into.

Other common times to experience strange moods are right after taking a nap, in the middle of the night— this is a very common time to experience anxiety and manic thoughts, as this is when adrenaline peaks in each 24-hour cycle—and right before bed. Bad moods right before bed usually mean that you stayed up too late, or are not sleeping enough. But there are plenty of people that also start to feel very stressed out and freezing cold right before bed as well (Wear Two Pairs of Socks to Bed Syndrome; WTPOSTBS), timed with the rise in aldosterone, another type of stress hormone, that starts to rise in the late evening. If that happens to you late at night, you guessed it—eat something!

Let's talk about some of these rhythms and fluctuations, because if we can level out these fluctuations our mood stability often follows suit.

Remember earlier when I said that going out in the natural light was inherently de-stressing? It is. In fact, natural outdoor light, even on a really cloudy day, is still a bajillion times more intense than even bright indoor lighting. Okay, my math isn't that precise, but outdoor light is significantly brighter. We all know that dark, cloudy days also have an impact on mood, and it's not for the better. The bright light of the full moon affects emotions. Suicide rates are typically higher in winter and higher in the high latitudes where there is less sunlight. Sun lamps and dawn-simulating alarm clocks (that use light to wake you up instead of sound) are proven to have benefits. We're highly affected by light. Dude, we're like moths.

And, we're affected by darkness. Darkness, while it happens every single day in most places, is actually a pretty tough biological challenge to face each night. During the night we are pounded with a barrage of stress hormones such as aldosterone, adrenaline, and finally cortisol which peaks right before the sun comes up. That's right—producing tons of stress hormones in your sleep! Hopefully now you're seeing why that whole sympathetic/parasympathetic thing is an oversimplification now. But hey, you're not reading this to become a scientist, but to improve your mood, so don't think too much.

The important thing to remember here is that, in a typical human with a relatively typical sleep schedule, you're going to see higher stress hormone levels in the middle of the night and morning, and then you'll see a steady reduction in stress hormones throughout the day. Finally, in early evening, the morning's stress hormones in the rearview mirror, you feel pretty good. Humans tend to feel so good in the early evening that body temperature, athletic performance, strength, and flexibility peak along with it. This feeling good isn't limited to physical attributes, but usually translates to significantly better mood stability and overall demeanor.

The question is, how do we win the battle against stress hormones and greater mood instability from late night to midday? For some, it's not an easy battle to win, and the battle happens each day with sluggishness, grogginess, moodiness, anxiety, irritability, greater coldness, more frequent urination, and general "pissy-ness" and blah. It's also much easier to get soul-suckingly depressed from morning to midday as well, especially if you don't get out into the natural light to start sobering up from your darkness hangover. And if you remain indoors watching television and moping about, good luck cheering up. You'll need it.

The real answer to how we win the battle is: We win it with food! What did you think I was going to say, St. John's Wort? Yeah right.

Food, outdoor light, maybe a little exercise while you're out there, and plenty of sleep the night before are the first answers. Meaningful, stimulating work is good also, but I'd still recommend moving your body around a little bit outdoors and getting your belly full of stress-lowering food first.

And what exactly is stress-lowering food? Stress-lowering foods, generally-speaking, are the S's: sugar, starch, salt, and saturated fat (although any fat will do, I mention saturated fat because most of my research and experience shows that it's superior for metabolism).

I don't think writing a whole cookbook to finish the book off is necessary to help guide you to these foods. These are the things that humans universally enjoy and that make food taste good, and they are things we downright crave when stressed or very hungry (same thing, basically). Be sure to get at least a little protein in there, too, to round out your otherwise carby meal. Carbohydrates in particular are fantastic at shutting down the sympathetic nervous system, especially when delivered in a calorie-dense and palatable package (fruit is not calorie dense!). The only problem with carbs is that they can sometimes cause a huge mood crash a couple hours after breakfast, but we'll get to that before all is said and done.

Paired with satisfying, filling, stick-to-your ribs food in the morning, you should also be cautious about consuming too many fluids if you find yourself having a mood crash with frequent urination a couple hours after breakfast each day. A lot of misguided people actually blame the carbohydrates themselves for causing this, even though carbohydrates often do not cause mood crash symptoms in the very same individual at any other time of day.

Hahahaha! Silly people. It's the hormones at that hour that cause drastic differences in glucose metabolism, fluid tolerance, and other things. That's a whole other tangent that I've already gone on elsewhere. No need to repeat it again here. Suffice it to say that it is possible for most people to dramatically improve this, and they should seek to improve it rather than avoid carbohydrates or food altogether during the high-stress morning hours. You can run from carbs, but you can't hide. And, interestingly, most can avoid the crash simply by consuming carbohydrates with a lower water content with additional salt. What is often dubbed anxiety and irritability-inducing "hypoglycemia" often has as much or more to do with fluids than it does carbohydrates. Try eating pancakes with syrup and well-salted eggs one morning with just a small beverage. The next day, just have the biggest smoothie you can stomach and nothing else.

Feel the profound differences in your mood and body temperature for the next several hours. If you're coming off a low-carb diet, you'll feel terrible with either breakfast. But it's not likely to last forever. Give your body at least a couple months to re-acclimate to carbs before blaming all your problems on them.

Keep that pee yellow through the mid-morning hours, and I bet you'll find a better mood corresponding with it. That includes you coffee drinkers so famous for peeing your brains out all morning. I'm not the caffeine police or anything. Just add lots of milk and sugar and even a pinch of salt to that coffee and consume it with food. Much better outcome several hours later. I can't promise you'll be "bulletproof" or anything, but you should feel greater mood stability.

Okay, I guess I covered the whole blood sugar thing enough to forego a separate section about it. If you want more information about the mid-morning "crash" that often triggers some nasty moods for you, my book *Hypoglycemia* focuses on that issue almost exclusively. It also contains less jackassery, which may be a plus if you're super annoyed with how this "book" is written at this point. I can't help it. I was victimized by collegiate education in creative writing. They taught me to express myself in creative and original ways. My grades weren't always the best.

Actually, I'm kind of in the "mood" to write some little essays on various mood-related topics from this point on. I might even put a revised version of an old blog post on serotonin in here as well. Kinda ghetto, but I can do whatever I want. I'm da boss.

Depression

As mentioned earlier, I'm verified by science to be the happiest human being alive. Here, I share all my secrets with you sorry lot of depressed whiners. Stop crying and pay attention.

I've never experiencing debilitating, chronic depression, but one thing I can do for sure is imagine it, because I've certainly experienced my fair share of horrible and inexplicable sadness. Fortunately for me, these episodes have always been brief—lasting from a few hours to a few days at the most. Then I'm all Mr. Smiley again unless that damn wifi router isn't working. Then lives are in danger.

There have been times where it has persisted longer but was not intense. The worst I've experienced was when living in Alaska. You would think it would be the winter that did me in, but I wasn't there in the winter. The month of September was enough to make me a wreck. I was living south of Ketchikan where it rains 140 inches per year, and if I'm not mistaken, September is one of the wettest months. It certainly was the summer I spent up there.

Every day was cold, wet, gray, windy, and 45 degrees. I was also trying to eat as little as possible, vowing not to eat a single cookie all month and often skipping breakfast (which makes it even harder to go face the cold elements). I was pretty perky earlier in the summer despite listening to too much Radiohead and Moby and being thousands of miles away from my girlfriend who had reported experimenting with not being my girlfriend while I was gone. I got up most days, went out hiking and fishing, and reeled in massive trout and salmon all morning before I reported to the kitchen to prepare dinner for the staff and guests. I don't remember crying over my girlfriend much when I was reeling in Sockeye salmon alongside of bears in streams that looked like the fishing scene in *The Sea Gypsies*.

But perky I was not when the sky turned gray and I got into the habit of sleeping in late—often not setting foot outdoors all day. I was miserable. Instead of waking up with a fish boner and even being excited about and enjoying my work, I started dreading it. Dreading getting out of bed even. Didn't even care about the salmon I had come so far to slay. Screw 'em. Screw everything.

I was super melancholy, so I listened to music I was in the mood for. More Radiohead on repeat, over and over again. Kid A and Hail to the Thief. Two of the most depressing albums of all time. This song makes Morrissey sound like New Kids on the Block. https://www.youtube.com/watch?v=U2taqRPi81E

The point of all this is quite simple. This depression felt completely circumstantial. I started feeling sorry for myself and feeling apathetic, but in reality it probably had little to do with any of the sad things I was thinking about. I was just thinking about sad things because of the combination of factors that all foster feelings of depression in susceptible individuals. And in response to the sadness, I did everything that a person could possibly do wrong in climbing my way out of it. I stayed in bed in a dark room with curtains pulled and no lights on. I didn't go outside. I didn't actively do or pursue anything. I listened to extremely emotional music with spellbinding, depressive melodies over and over again. I ate as little as possible, particularly yummy sweet things that I've always had a strong affinity for. I avoided social encounters.

Thankfully for me, the lodge closed for the season at the end of the month, and I got the hell out of there and dove into a totally new set of habits and rhythms once I did. Adios depression.

I understand that it's not always this simple to churn your way out of depression. For many, no matter how many tanning excursions to the beach and fishing trips they go on or social interaction they get, no matter how much peppy, pop music they listen to, and no matter what amount of carbs sweet carbs they ingest—nothing will lead to resolution of their deep, dark, dreary, disorder. I'm not suggesting that the cure is simple for everyone. But for some, it is. And for the rest, observance of smart practices that keep mood from tumbling into the abyss of sadness should be prioritized anyhow.

Here is a concise list of what I've found to be the most helpful for myself, and what has also been responsible for the greatest mood enhancement in my readers and clients over the past few years:

1. **Eat enough.** Our bodies and minds are not designed to be satisfied when we're underfed. Of all foods, carbohydrates are the most important for mood enhancement. Be very careful about restricting them, even if it seems to stabilize your mood at first, results in weight loss, or other seductive traps. And morning is the most important time to eat. Skipping breakfast and pigging out late at night is more of the eating pattern I associate with depression.

2. **Sleep enough.** We're also not designed to be happy when we're short on sleep. There has been some information that has surfaced recently about the use of sleep restriction, fasting, and other stress-inducers for relieving depression. It's true that a good surge of stress hormones can feel like a cup of coffee and provide a jolt in mood and energy. This is not a smart, long-term, holistic approach. You need sleep. 8-10 hours per day ideally. Work on finding a solution that doesn't involve undersleeping.

3. **Wake up at dawn.** Unless you have to work late and cannot go to bed at least eight hours prior to dawn, try your best to get your body conditioned

to waking up when all other diurnal creatures do. Waking up early must work to make you happy or all farmers would have shot themselves by now. That's science bro.

4. **Get outside as fast as you can.** Don't hurt yourself running down any stairs or anything, but you would be wise to get out of your house and into the sunlight as quickly as you can. Not only is bright light an essential vitamin for improving mood, but your home or apartment is like a big nest for you to lay a depression egg in. Stay away from the nest as much as possible. There are also other compelling reasons to get outside if you suffer from depression aside from the bright light, such as negative ions and reduced exposure to electrical activity in the home.

5. **Dive into something productive.** Doing nothing and being aimless is a powerful depression trigger. And once the depressive feelings set in, forget about it. It's a downward spiral from there. I mean, who feels like getting out of the house, working on a project, or doing some pushups when you're depressed? Yes, doing some physical activity counts as doing something productive. It probably deserves its very own number, as it can be very powerful. But yeah, do something productive if possible. Something mentally or physically stimulating. I don't know about you, but without physical activity and/or lots of cool projects to keep me busy I'm a total mess.

6. **Create a routine.** I want to punch myself in the face for even saying that, as I'm the most lousy routine-keeper ever, but routines are powerfully beneficial. It allows you to do stuff that you know keeps you feeling and functioning your best emotionally and otherwise without even having to think about or analyze it. You just do it habitually and automatically as part of the template for your day. I'm not saying to become a droid, but forming new habits that include some of the items on this list are a powerful defense against the doldrums.

7. **Be social.** Like in real life, not just the internet. Again, pot calling the kettle black here, but social interaction with others is incredibly valuable (I hear). Of course, when you're depressed you don't feel like being social. It might be better to work some social interaction into your routines on some kind of schedule. You know, Monday night football with Bob. Mancala hour on Tuesdays. Salsa dancing on Wednesday. Stuff like that only cooler, so you don't shoot yourself in the face. Mancala hour? Yeah, that's not worth living for.

8. **Go easy on the Morrissey.** Man I love Morrissey. And my restraint from listening to melancholy music is pretty pitiful. I'm listening to Radiohead right now after writing about them earlier. I think I gravitate to that type of music because I do have those tendencies to feel achy longings for that untouchable something out there in the cosmos. Fortunately I'm not at a very depressed point in my life. I don't even listen to music that much to be

honest. I'm constantly around my girlfriend and her daughter, and melancholy music doesn't fly. But there's no question that, if you're battling depression, you should use music to make you feel better, not dig yourself deeper. Listen to something that makes you mad, happy, energized—anything but more depressed.

9. **Reduce screen time.** While I could go on a big tangent about brain waves and television and try to make a big case here, I think the most important thing about reducing screen time is that television, phones, tablets, and computers hinder your ability to follow through on just about every anti-depression intervention I've listed here! Seriously! Electronics are the eternal foe of productivity, leaving the home, getting enough sleep, being social, exercising, and more. At the very least, try to start your day away from the screen and come back to it later once you've followed through on your more invigorating, inspiring habits.

10. **And to quote another 80's movie, "And from now on, stop playing with yourself."** I don't know if that will really help or not, but it's not a real self-esteem enhancer. Mostly I included this to score points with my girlfriend. She's like the masturbation police.

Again, this may be yet another set of tips that seem idiotic in their simplicity. A person with depression may even feel insulted by these simple suggestions. These are almost common sense, and I can't imagine many disagreeing with more than a couple items on this list. Again, I'm not saying that in these ten items lies a universal cure for all cases of depression. But if it was me, and I was facing a serious mood disorder, you can be sure that I would ace every item on that list before reaching for the Prozac or a similar SSRI (Selective Serotonin Reuptake Inhibitor). Because as you're about to read, the famous "happy chemical" has a sadder side.

The Sadder Side of Serotonin

Are you sad? Depressed? Tired? Crave them evil #$%#ohydrates? Well hell son you just need you some serotonin! Serotonin makes you happy! Whee!!!

No book about mood would be complete without a mention about serotonin, but you're about to hear some things about serotonin that don't jive with the vibe you may have gotten about it from drug commercials. I just said "jive" and "vibe" in the same sentence in case you didn't notice.

The research and cultural status quo on serotonin doesn't make much sense, and is full of contradiction. Strangely, everyone seems to be madly in love with serotonin (people even have tattoos celebrating it—I hope they don't read this!) and is fully satisfied with the label of "happy juice." Serotonin makes you happy, everyone seems to believe, and if you aren't happy then well, let's figure out how to get more serotonin in ya. Buck up little camper, we'll beat that slump, together.

When everyone in the media, in the health field, and beyond start to collectively believe in a very simple and narrow story about any one thing, you can probably be sure that some kind of Scientific Sasquatch has come into being. The belief that serotonin is like the biochemical equivalent of Happy Gilmore sharing a Happy Meal with a bunch of Care Bears in heaven holding hands and skipping with Mr. Rogers and Bob Ross is not just Kardashingly shallow. It's criminally inaccurate.

In pursuit of maintaining good mitochondrial respiration and keeping metabolism from declining with age, in pursuit of squelching stress hormone production and keeping the anabolic hormones of youth in full swing, and in pursuit of minimizing inflammation and more—what science increasingly leads us towards when it comes to the prevention and cure of the modern world's most common illnesses, the recruitment of serotonin in that fight is about as productive as (insert clever, sarcastic metaphor).

What I'm really getting at is that serotonin sucks, in a general sense. And what people think about serotonin—in terms of how to raise it, what it will do for you when it rockets up, and so forth are really kinda dumb and poorly thought out. But it doesn't take a whole lot of research to determine that serotonin isn't all it's cracked up to be, and that those who think it's going to cure everything from depression to seasonal affective disorder and help you shed some pounds while you're at it are some pretty confused people with a very superficial understanding of the many things that serotonin regulates in the brain and body.

Let's discuss six sad things about serotonin:

1. **Serotonin is highly involved in hibernation, lowering body temperature and more.** It rises as daylight shortens and helps to trigger many of the metabolic changes that occur with hibernating animals—all of which are synonymous with a reduced metabolic rate, reduced respiratory rate, increased insulin resistance, reduced carbon dioxide levels, reduced energy level, reduced body temperature, increased histamine, reduced peristalsis, and so forth— just to name a few. If those things were good, we would get progressively healthier with advancing age. But they aren't, and we don't. Those are all biomarkers of poorer health, lower vitality levels, and increasing risk of degenerative disease.

2. **Serotonin is fattening and triggers insulin resistance.** Knowing serotonin's role in hibernation, it should come as no surprise that "antidepressant" drugs like Prozac, which increase serotonin levels through sort of a recycling process, are very fattening and known to dramatically increase the risk of developing type 2 diabetes. Wow. Real shocker there. Increase the levels of a substance that makes you tired and want to sleep all the time and induces weight gain and insulin resistance… And watch it cause weight gain and insulin resistance!

3. **Serotonin plays a primary role in seasonal affective disorder (SAD).** There is a great deal of shocking bull$#@^ when it comes to seasonal affective disorder, as the bass ackwards rumor that seasonal affective disorder has something to do with decreasing levels of serotonin is pervasive, yet increasing darkness and shortened day length causes INCREASES in serotonin, and increases in laying around all day— lifeless, sad, and wanting to shoot your Alaskan self in the ear in early January. Oh yeah, "sunlight raises serotonin" says the brainwashed serotonin lovers. That must be why serotonin peaks at midnight when the sun is really shining bright! Both high-powered lights in the morning as well as negative ions have been shown to be effective treatments for seasonal affective disorder, which is interesting when you consider the quote coming up in #4...

4. **Serotonin causes depression**. I was perusing through a pro-serotonin article and found this contradictory gem lying there, plucked from a book on controlling asthma (more on that in a sec). It says a lot, and is probably part of the reason why I have always found failure to make it outdoors by about 10am to be extremely depressing (modern dwellings are notoriously high in positive ions, which raise serotonin)...

"Research by Dr. Leslie Hawkins at the University of Surrey, UK, showed that levels of the hormone serotonin in the blood, brain and other tissues seemed to be reduced by negative ions. Serotonin is a substance that plays a part in brain chemistry, and imbalances in it lead to depression and other mental disturbances. Dr.

Hawkins suggested that air rich in negative ions has a stimulating effect while too many positive ions, and thus high levels of serotonin in the body, are depressing. This may explain why ionisers help in cases of irritability and stress."

5. **Serotonin exacerbates and may even cause asthma**. That should be no surprise seeing that serotonin is synonymous with reduced carbon dioxide levels, constricts bronchioles, plays a role in the general inflammatory response (stimulating the pituitary gland), and so forth. It would also make sense that if negative ions decrease seasonal affective disorder that they would also reduce asthma symptoms if the cause (high serotonin) was the same, which they of course do (negative ions reducing asthma symptoms, that is).

6. **Serotonin may play a causal role in schizophrenia, autism, and countless other neurological disorders**. The bulk of our serotonin supply is produced in the digestive tract. Serotonin increases with digestive distress. Serotonin forms somewhat of a vicious cycle with the digestive tract. Serotonin suppresses metabolism, suppressed metabolism fosters the overgrowth of yeast and bacteria in the small intestine, which in turn produces a much greater outpouring of serotonin produced in the gut, especially when "health" food like whole grains, legumes, nuts, seeds, and raw fruits and vegetables are consumed. Dr. Natasha Campbell-McBride's *Gut and Psychology Syndrome* (GAPS), a theory that groups many psychological disorders and pins it on digestive

abnormalities is most likely related to the increased serotonin activity with impaired digestion.

This is just a short list of course. Serotonin is involved in the general disease, aging, inflammation, and degeneration process—from hypertension to asthma to schizophrenia to insomnia to diabetes to depression—of which there is tremendous overlap and redundancy between all of them, them, them. The list easily could have been titled "66 Sad Things About Serotonin."

If you see lots of authors, researchers, and even formal studies that seem to contradict what was said here, keep looking, look carefully, and review the breadth of what you find only after thoroughly taking in a comprehensive viewpoint—keeping in mind that Selective Serotonin Reuptake Inhibitors (SSRI) drugs are some of the top selling drugs on earth, and that the pharmaceutical industry is the primary financier of medical research, medical education, and the media empires that have hardwired you to believe that serotonin is great stuff, and if you are sad or anxious or tired you need more of it.

At the very least, be a little more cautious before reaching for SSRI's, tryptophan, 5-HTP, and melatonin (a related chemical) pills if your mood is off. Make sure to master the fundamentals before you take that leap. If you're already taking these substances, be careful about coming off of them, which can also be dangerous if your mood disorders are severe.

For further geekage, listen to Josh and Jeanne Rubin's interview with Ray Peat on serotonin (http://bit.ly/1y1hQV5), and some of the links below that provide some validation to the claims made in this chapter.

- Serotonin and Asthma (http://bit.ly/1w1jCWE)
- Serotonin and Hypertension (http://bit.ly/1w1jCWE)
- Hibernation and Insulin Resistance (http://1.usa.gov/1rELYPY)
- SSRI's Increase Diabetes Risk (http://bit.ly/11CrT62)
- Serotonin and Schizophrenia (http://bit.ly/1uTDZi9)
- Serotonin and Autism (http://bit.ly/12dassF)
- Serotonin and IQ, ADD, ADHD, Downs Syndrome, Depression (http://bit.ly/124rTfU)
- Asthma and Positive and Negative Ions (http://bit.ly/1w1mcMt)
- Bright Lights and Negative Ions for Winter Depression (http://bit.ly/12daS2r)
- Serotonin and Hibernation (http://bit.ly/1rEOh5J)
- Dawn Stimulation and Ionizers for Seasonal Affective Disorder (http://bit.ly/1tz1Lzx)
- Negative Ions Lower Serotonin (http://bit.ly/1y1jPbL)
- Histamine and Serotonin in Hibernation (http://bit.ly/1z2uDVy)

- Ionizers as an Anti-Depressant
  (http://bit.ly/1vWMZda)
- Serotonin, Aggression, and Depression
  (http://bit.ly/1zFlPVt)
- Tryptophan, Serotonin, and Aging
  (http://bit.ly/1xTl9cT)

Grain Brain

With the increasing popularity of bashing grains, it would be out of character for me to remain silent in a book having something to do with cognitive function.

Believe me, I'm perfectly aware of every single point that Dr. Perlmutter makes in his book *Grain Brain*. I've followed the alternative health and nutrition movement for almost a solid decade, and I've received a massive overdose of grain phobia coming at me from all sides in the process. While I was eager to join the bandwagon at first, as my research progressed, and as I stumbled upon more and more empty promises and sciencey-sounding theories that turned out to have no basis in reality, I became increasingly capable of separating the wheat from the chaff so-to-speak.

So what are grains, gluten, and all these carbohydrates doing to our brains, emotions, pleasure centers, etc.? Are they making us all crazy? Are they the primary nutritional cause of neurodegeneration? Do they create greater blood sugar and mood instability? Should we avoid them?

First of all, no health question should ever be posed with the word "we." Health information and dietary decisions are entirely individual matters. I know some people who break out into rashes, ache all over, and have massive anxiety attacks when they eat so much as a slice of toast. I've also helped hundreds of people recover their health in incalculable ways, and climb out from scary, debilitated places, by ditching a gluten-free diet and religiously eating pancakes for breakfast daily.

Personally, I improved my mood tremendously several years ago when I began eating lots of carbohydrates again—primarily in the form of tubers and grains. It also did wonders for my digestion, as I had suffered through years of intense heartburn after every meal when grains were limited in my diet. My girlfriend at the time had developed an autoimmune disease during her stint on a low-carbohydrate diet, and after resuming the consumption of some of her favorite foods like bread and crackers, the autoimmune disease completely vanished and has never returned. My current girlfriend was able to completely stabilize her epilepsy with what I jokingly referred to as "The French Toast Cure" several years ago. Prior to that, her epilepsy and OCD was severe enough that she had to quit her job. White flour to the rescue!

There were other factors at play in all of those scenarios of course, and for long-term health and overall nutrition one could hardly call French toast and pancakes optimal foods, but the fact of the matter remains: I've seen far too many people develop the problems gluten is supposed to cause on a grain-free diet and too many people recover from those problems by adding grains back into their diets to swallow the anti-gluten Kool-Aid.

I poured some into my mouth, but I did not swallow!

Being perfectly frank, nothing in the health and nutrition world is as bad as it is made out to be or as good as it is made out to be. With the infinite mountain of data and studies, anyone can build a case against pretty much anything, and at the end of it all make some sense and have apparent "evidence" with which to back up their claims. Unfortunately, nothing about this is scientific or science. It seems the world is currently very confused about this, as taking an isolated research paper or study out of context and making a claim based on its findings is considered legitimate evidence. It's not. And usually the ones that are doing this are doing so to make a big splash on the web, in the media, or in their books. It's one of the major reasons we're all so confused, and how the research currently available to us all can be bent and twisted in so many ways. Like a pretzel. Mmmm, pretzels.

For example, take the common trend en vogue today of calling sugar "addictive." It activates the same region of the brain and causes the release of the same neurotransmitters as ingesting cocaine or other addictive substances. Therefore, sugar is proven to be addictive.

It's very compelling and hard to argue against. Is it true? Of course not. Sugar addictive? Please. It's no more addictive than pizza or bacon or potato chips or cheese. It's no more addictive than sex or showering or shopping or drinking a glass of water when you're thirsty or a hug. Fact of the matter is that we have pleasure centers in our brain that guide us towards things we need. The more we are in need of something, the more our pleasure centers do backflips. I've been "addicted" to raw, dry oats before when I was literally on the brink of starvation. Almost everything we do that we find enjoyable lights up our pleasure centers at varying intensities. It's proof of nothing.

Let's take another example as it pertains to wheat and gluten specifically. This supposedly "scientific" belief is pervasive to a certain segment of the health and nutrition scene. And boy is it ever a "scene." The belief is that ingesting wheat causes an increase in advanced glycation end products (AGES) in the brain. Advanced glycation end products, they assert, are formed when glucose and proteins form these nasty AGES. To prevent these from forming, the solution is to prevent rises in blood sugar by avoiding the overconsumption of carbohydrates, particularly wheat because it registers at the top of the glycemic index—meaning that blood sugar rises faster when consuming wheat than nearly all foods.

It sounds pretty reasonable on the surface, and with a neurologist like Perlmutter to back it up, how can it be wrong? But dig deeper and you'll see that there are incredible leaps in logic to go from point A to point Z in this entrenched facet of low-carbolatry.

The whole theory is based on the idea that high blood sugar increases glycation. It does. I have my doubts that it is the greatest contributor to the formation of AGES after my studies into the role that polyunsaturated fats play in this process, but I'll still give it to them. However, wheat doesn't cause high blood sugar. It may cause blood sugar to temporarily rise, but it doesn't cause chronic elevations in blood sugar. In fact, a comprehensive look into the matter, and more importantly, actual experience in working with dozens of individuals, myself included, to lower fasting and postprandial glucose levels (I once got my own fasting level to 67 mg/dl with postprandial readings at only 75 mg/dl)—carbohydrates clearly play a vital role in improving glucose clearance and glucose metabolism in general.

No wonder this observation was made by Denis Burkitt several decades ago:

"It is of interest that diets high in fibre-rich cereals and tuberous vegetables tend to result in an improvement in basal blood glucoses."

Burkitt, Denis, Hugh Trowell, and Kenneth Heaton. *Dietary Fibre, Fibre-Depleted Foods and Disease.* Academic Press: London, 1985, p. 281.

Take a look at a real case study with a real human being adding high-glycemic starchy foods back into her diet, including grains. The decrease in insulin and blood sugar levels are astounding:

http://180degreehealth.com/starch-lowers-insulin/

Now, if rises in blood sugar following the ingestion of high-glycemic carbohydrates like wheat and potatoes actually lowers total blood sugar and improves glycemic control, this whole theory of carbs equals high blood sugar equals AGES equals neurodegenerative disease falls completely on its face. It may even be completely backwards. Most likely, it's just focused on the wrong perpetrator. They should be focusing on what causes a disruption to insulin sensitivity and glucose clearance, and that is certainly not wheat, gluten, or any kind of carbohydrate.

I don't mean to write an entire thesis on the factual errors and leaps in logic that occur in some of the more popular anti-wheat tomes that have torn the book market to shreds in recent years. The purpose in writing this is just to relieve you of a sliver of the brainwashing you might have received, and to become a little less convinced that various popular diet authors are preaching the absolute, unshakeable truth. They aren't. The ones on the biggest and loudest crusades are usually the most egregious scientists of them all. The good scientists are quietly pondering and treating their ideas and hypotheses very tentatively—taking all the viewpoints into consideration and avoiding jumping to conclusions with great discipline and integrity.

Anyway, the point of all this really is to shine some light on the validity of the anti-wheat craze. Is it justified? Has it been taken too far?

No, it's not justifiable, and yes, it has been taken way too far. Should you avoid grains? I would wholeheartedly recommend doing some experimentation with a grain-free diet if you have severe mood stability problems. I find that wheat does in fact cause slightly more mood instability personally, but certainly not enough to justify the difficulty in complete abstinence. Plus, when I do abstain from grains completely, I have a really tough time consuming adequate calories to support a high metabolic rate, and then even more problems creep in—mood-wise and beyond. But what matters here is that I was able to figure this out for myself with honest assessments and open-minded curiosity. You can do the same and come up with a pretty decent custom-built diet all on your own. Just be careful of falling for the honeymoon effect. If it feels too good to be true, it probably is.

Is there legitimacy to the whole gluteomorphines and stuff? A little bit, but again, it's been blown out of proportion, and everyone who's ever had a headache or a mood swing is now thinking it was caused by this metabolite or whatever.

The point is that you should experiment freely, and that you should always view someone that sounds like a crusader as a charlatan. They probably are, as health and nutrition matters are too complex to possibly be that sure of THE answer. I know because I used to be a charlatan myself, but have backed way down since I matured enough to see the errors in my immature thinking. Now my thinking is much more mature. I don't think I've mentioned my testicles a single time in this entire book.

And you know, between the call to experiment freely and the mention of my balls, it's probably a good ending point. Nothing I could say from this point forward could top that combination of awesomeness.

Conclusion

So that's it? No elaborate discussions about amino acids, B vitamins, or herbal remedies? No special diets, South American superfoods, or meal plans?

Sorry. It's those damn, basic, boring fundamentals that everyone forgets again. Eat well, sleep well, don't do drugs, go outside, be social, exercise, get up early, eat a good breakfast, and pee yellow.

As I've mentioned several times already, the point of this book is not necessarily to function as a cure-all for any and every mood disorder under the sun (although getting under the sun is the closest thing there is to a cure-all). Its purpose is to point out that the cause of your issues may be much simpler than you think and easier to fix than you think as well. This book is meant to be a starting point for those that are concerned about their emotional health, as well as a refocusing manual for those that have desperately pursued exotic cures and torturous diets to no avail.

If you implement the strategies discussed in this book with gusto, and at the end of it all you still feel like the root of your problems aren't physical—but have much more to do with a variety of traumas you've experienced in the past and present—I would strongly encourage you to pursue the work of Bella Dodds. You can start with reading her book on anxiety specifically, which lays the foundation for her approach to resolving any mood disorder. It's called, simply, The Anxiety Solution.

Bella and I originally planned to co-author a book on anxiety together, but decided near the end that our separate approaches and completely different writing styles shouldn't be meshed together in the same book. It was the right call. I mean, I don't think she makes any 80's references at all!

May your fingers and toes always be warm and your pee be yellow, your breathing calm and your mood mellow.

Now go have a wonderful day. There's plenty of sunshine headed your way. Zip-a-dee-do-da n' shit.

Raising Metabolism eCourse

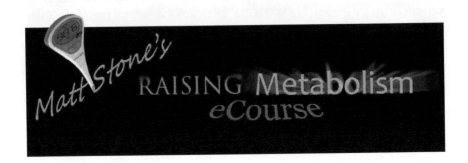

Obviously I have a little bit of a thing for this metabolism stuff. I don't mean to sound like a charlatan, but let me put it to you this way. If you have health problems—including those of the emotional variety—and you have any symptoms of a low metabolism including a low resting body temperature (below 98 degrees F or 37 degrees C), the first thing you should do before trying anything else is spend some time getting your metabolic rate up to snuff. It's a positive health investment for everyone, and many ailments are impossible to eliminate without restoring proper metabolic function—which influences every single biochemical reaction that takes place in the human body.

I created the Raising Metabolism eCourse as a way to start at the beginning and go through the entire educational process of understanding why it's important, how it gets screwed up, and precisely how to go about fixing it. It's completely free, delivered to your email inbox over a period of 90 days, thorough, and complete.

Sign up for it, and you'll also get all of my new book releases for free and probably all of my old ones at some point, too. I'm a sucker. I'll do anything for you. Just love me!

To sign up, go to www.180degreehealth.com and follow the simple instructions.

Please Review This!

I hope you enjoyed this short book and, at the very least, are more focused on the basic fundamentals of good self-care in approaching your health problems big and small, physical and emotional.

If this book helped or at least entertained you in any way, all I ask in return is that you take a moment to write an honest, sincere review of this book on Amazon. It will only take a few minutes, and it would help me out more than you can imagine.

About the Author

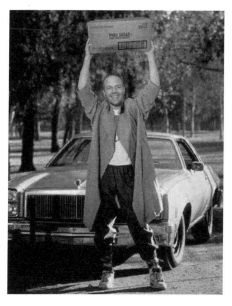

"With a high metabolic rate, EVERYTHING works better."

Matt Stone is an independent health researcher, #1 Amazon bestselling author of way too many books, and the founder of 180DegreeHealth, a controversial website that has challenged the status quo on health with a combination of cutting-edge science, radical common sense, and gratuitous 80's references since 2006.

In his most popular books, *Eat for Heat* and the *Diet Recovery* series, Stone lays out explicit instructions for achieving a high metabolic rate, the details of which are Stone's greatest discovery in his decade of intensive research.

With an increase in metabolic rate, thousands of Stone's readers and clients have reported improvements in a vast array of disorders: constipation, hair loss, low libido, acid reflux, insomnia, anxiety, cold hands and feet, frequent urination, allergies, skin conditions, chronic infections, infertility, and countless others, all while eating common, enjoyable, comfort foods to their heart's content.

To learn more, start by signing up for the FREE 90-Day Raising Metabolism eCourse at www.180degreehealth.com.

Made in the USA
Middletown, DE
05 February 2015